Take Care of Yourself

Caring for Your Teeth

by Mari Schuh

PEBBLE
a capstone imprint

Published by Pebble, an imprint of Capstone.
1710 Roe Crest Drive, North Mankato, Minnesota 56003
capstonepub.com

Library of Congress Cataloging-in-Publication Data
Names: Schuh, Mari C., 1975- author.
Title: Caring for your teeth / by Mari Schuh.
Description: North Mankato, Minnesota : Pebble, [2022] | Series: Take care of yourself | Includes bibliographical references and index. | Audience: Ages 5-8 | Audience: Grades K-1 | Summary: "A healthy mouth is more than just a beautiful smile. Readers learn how to care for their teeth, foods to eat for healthy teeth, and what to avoid so they don't damage their teeth"— Provided by publisher.
Identifiers: LCCN 2021029829 (print) | LCCN 2021029830 (ebook) | ISBN 9781663976819 (hardcover) | ISBN 9781666326673 (paperback) | ISBN 9781666326680 (pdf) | ISBN 9781666326703 (kindle edition)
Subjects: LCSH: Teeth—Care and hygiene—Juvenile literature.
Classification: LCC RK63 .S3824 2022 (print) | LCC RK63 (ebook) | DDC 617.6/01—dc23
LC record available at https://lccn.loc.gov/2021029829
LC ebook record available at https://lccn.loc.gov/2021029830

Image Credits
Capstone Studio: Karon Dubke, 9, 13, 14, 17, 19; Dreamstime: James Boardman, 7; Shutterstock: Anna Golant (design element) throughout, Artem Sokolov, 10didesign021, 5, Elovich, 20, GIOck, 20, Monkey Business Images, 15, Odua Images, cover, RACOBOVT, 21, Sergey Novikov, 18, View-point, 20, wong sze yuen, 11, wowowG, 6

Editorial Credits
Editor: Erika L. Shores; Designer: Heidi Thompson; Media Researcher: Jo Miller; Production Specialist: Tori Abraham

Printed in the United States   5155

Table of Contents

Words in **bold** are in the glossary.

Your Teeth

Have you brushed your teeth today?
Did you remember to use **floss**? Caring
for your teeth is an important way to stay
healthy. It helps you have a healthy life.

Your teeth help you in many ways.
You use your teeth to talk. They help you
chew food. Healthy teeth help you feel good.

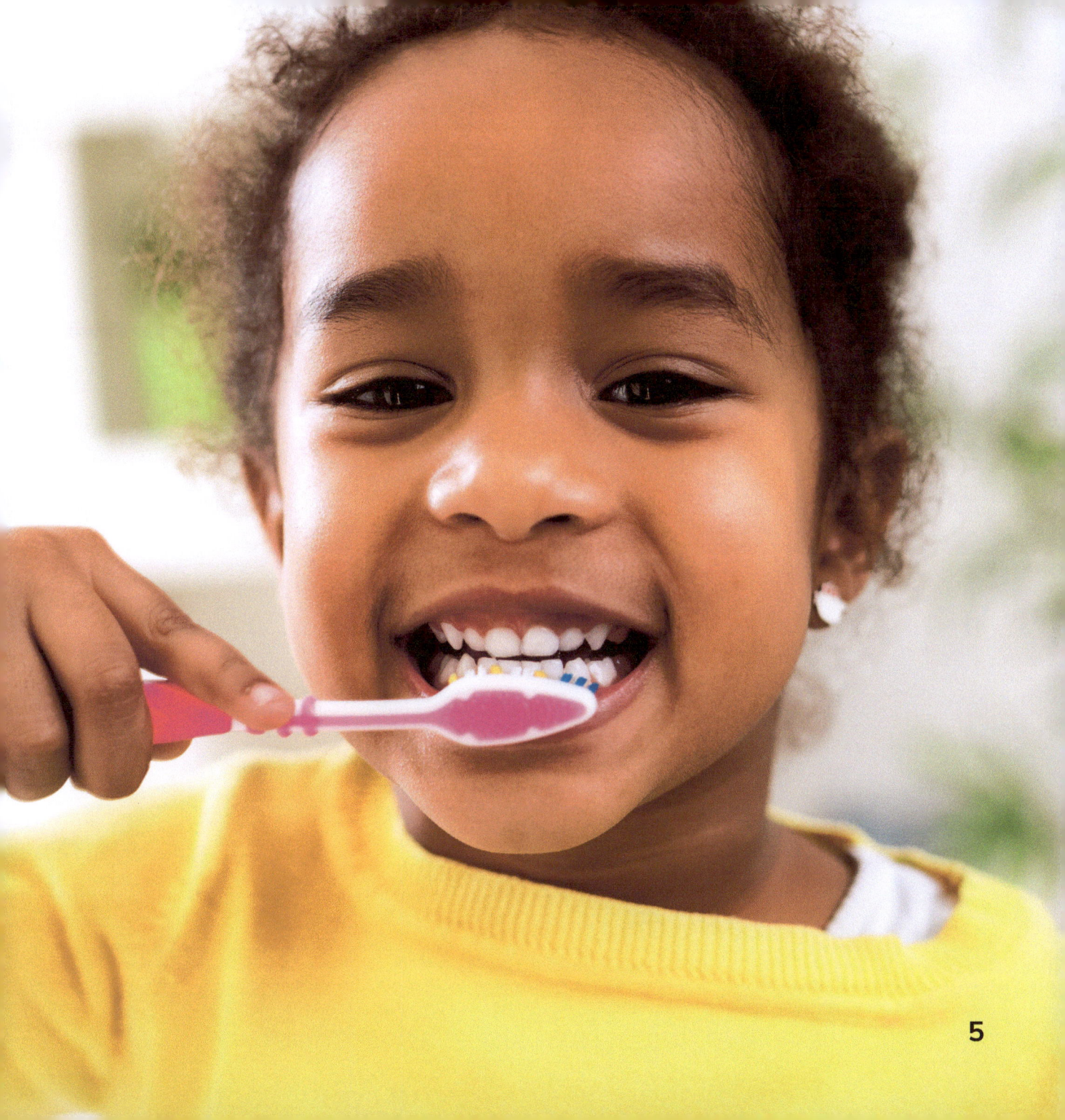

Healthy and Safe

Make sure to take good care of your teeth. This can keep you from having tooth problems. **Plaque** can form on teeth. This can cause tooth decay. Then you might get a **cavity**.

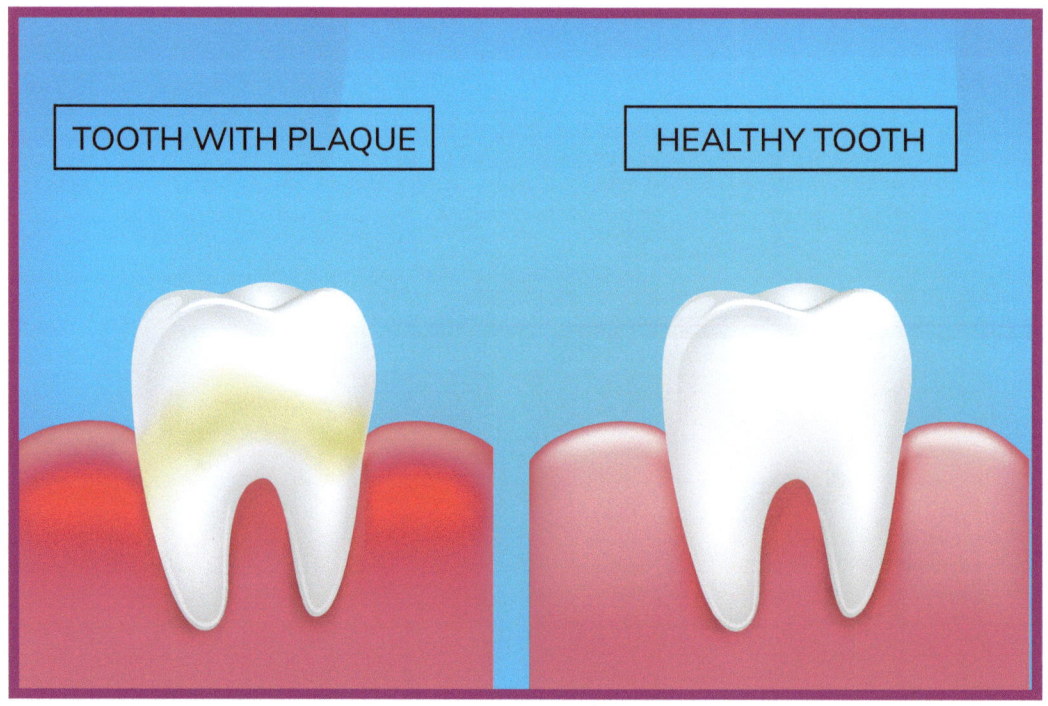

TOOTH WITH PLAQUE

HEALTHY TOOTH

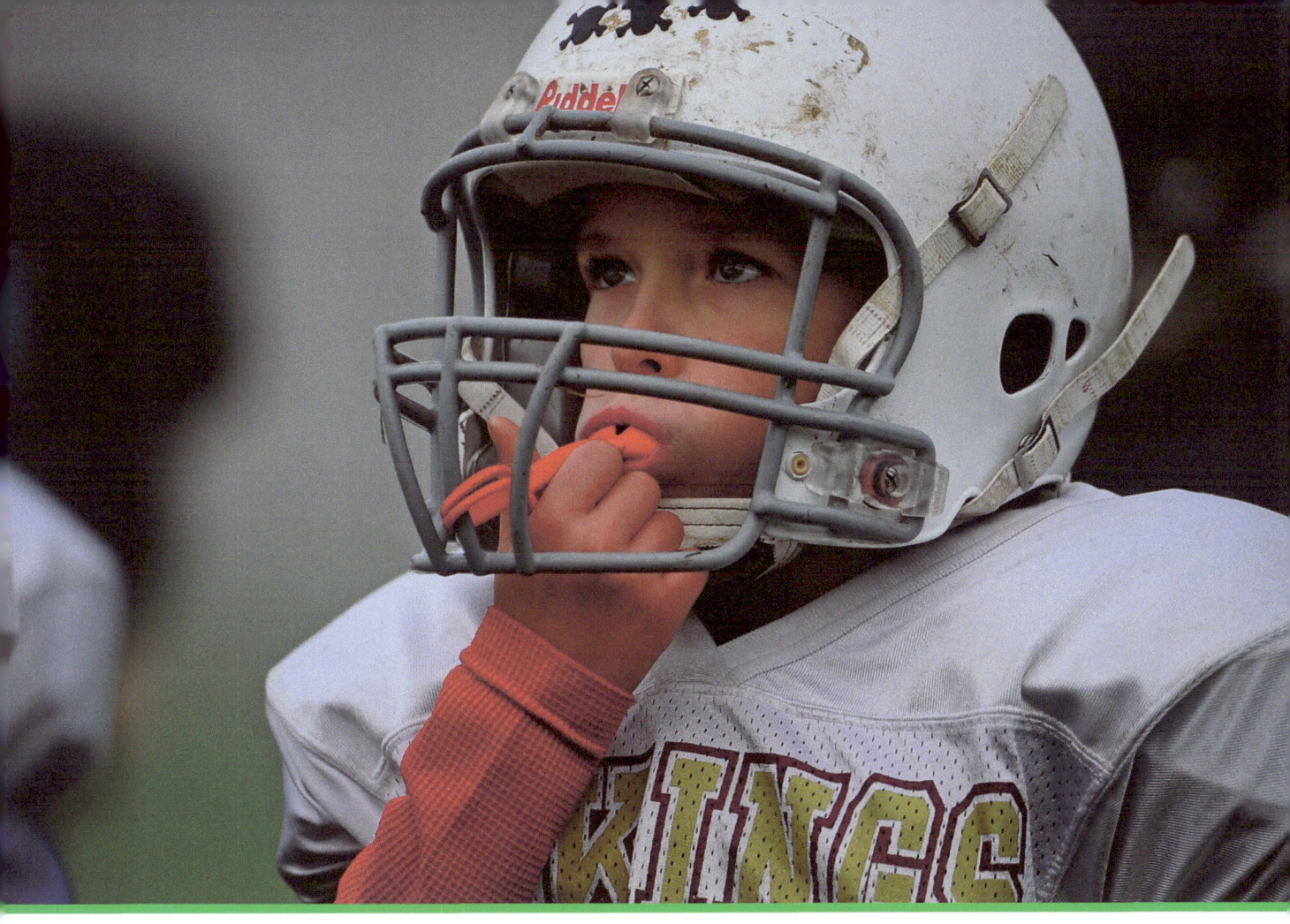

Protect your teeth. Wear a mouth guard
when you play sports. Don't use your teeth
to open up things. Use scissors instead.
If your teeth hurt, tell a grown-up.

Get Ready to Brush

Brushing your teeth keeps them clean. Brush after you eat breakfast. Also brush before you go to bed. Too tired at bedtime? Then try to brush a little earlier.

Pick a fun toothbrush with soft bristles. Be sure to use a toothpaste with **fluoride**. How much toothpaste do you need? Not much. The size of a pea or bean is enough.

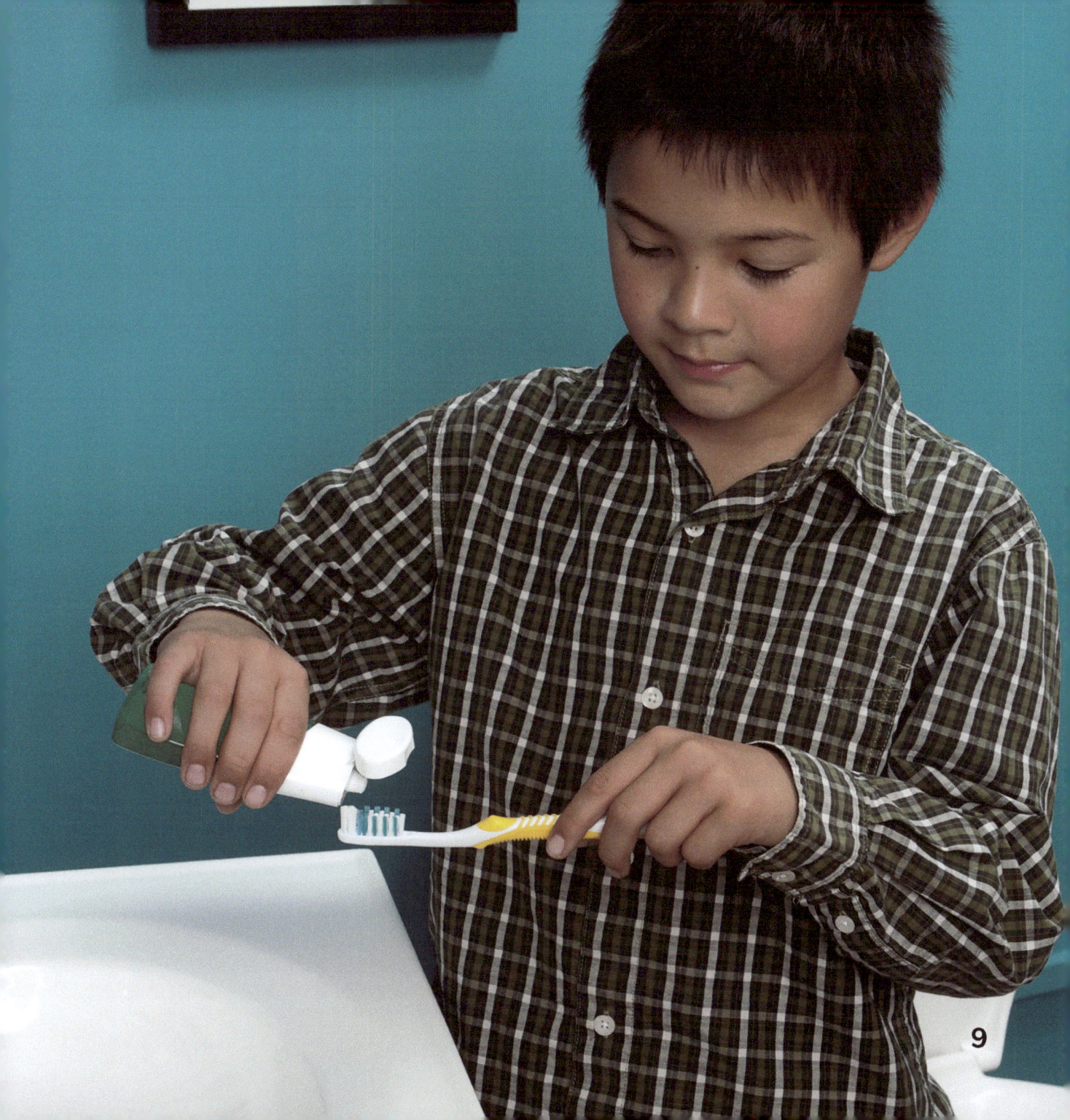

9

How to Brush

Gently brush each tooth. Brush all sides of your teeth. Brush in small circles. You should brush for two minutes or more. Don't rush. Use a timer. Or listen to a song while you brush.

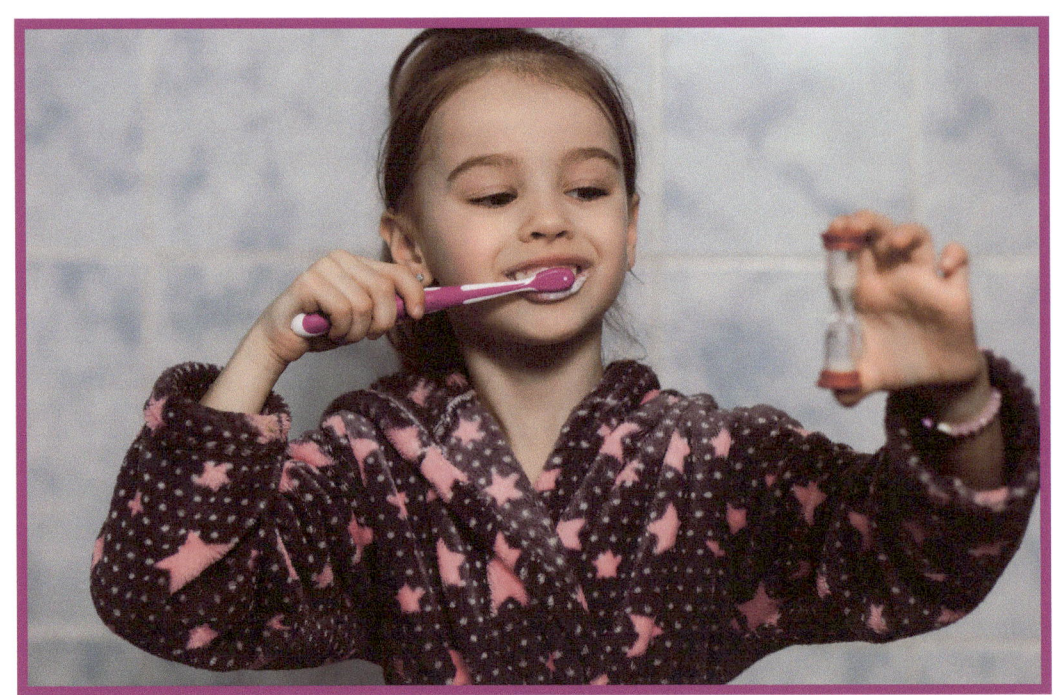

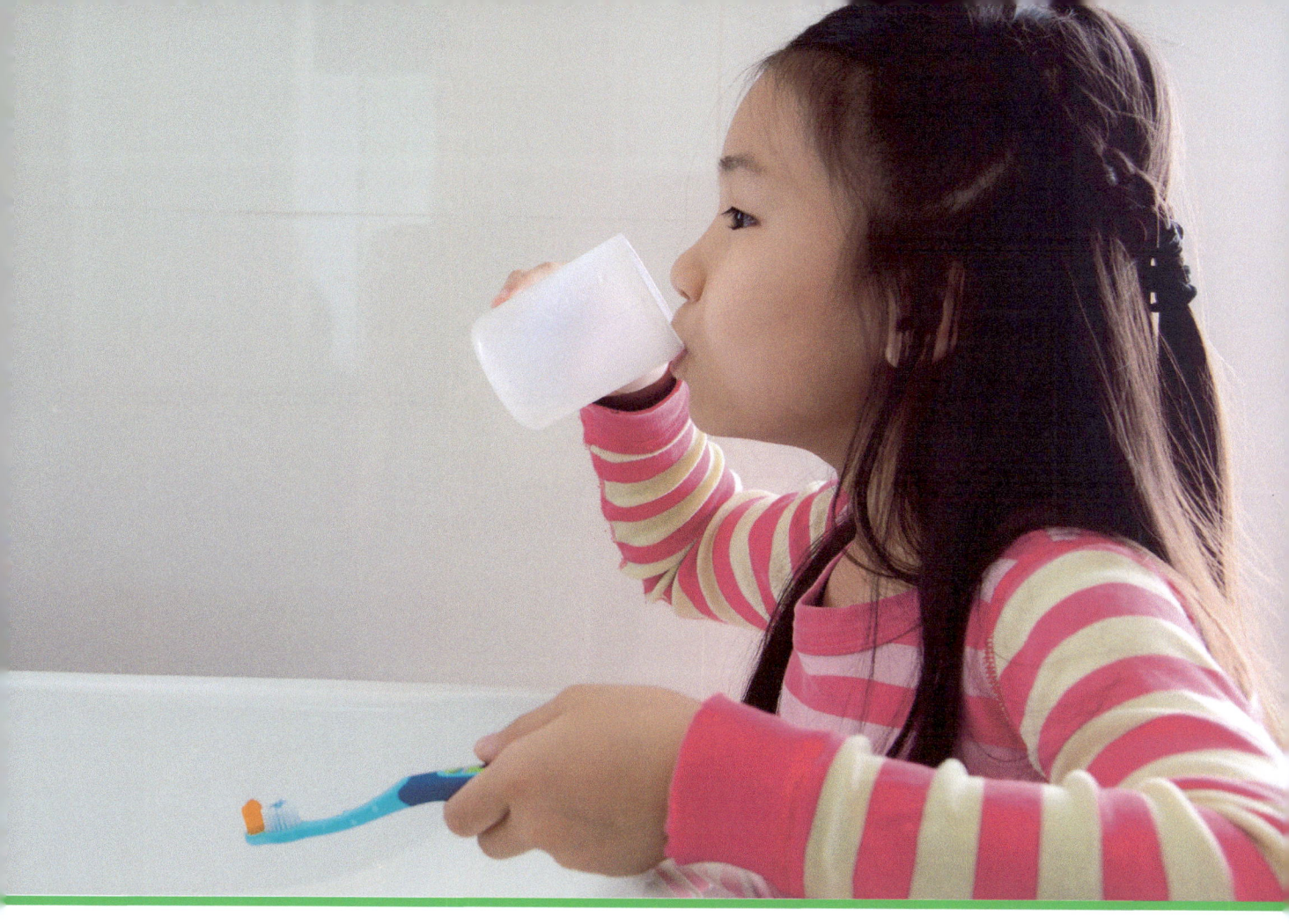

Brush your **gums** too. You can even brush
your tongue. All done? Be sure to spit out your
toothpaste. Some people add one more step.
They rinse their mouth with mouthwash.

Flossing

Brushing isn't the only step to healthy teeth. Flossing is important too! Use dental floss to clean between your teeth. This gets rid of food stuck in your teeth.

Use floss once a day. Slide the floss between each tooth along your gums. Gently move the floss back and forth.

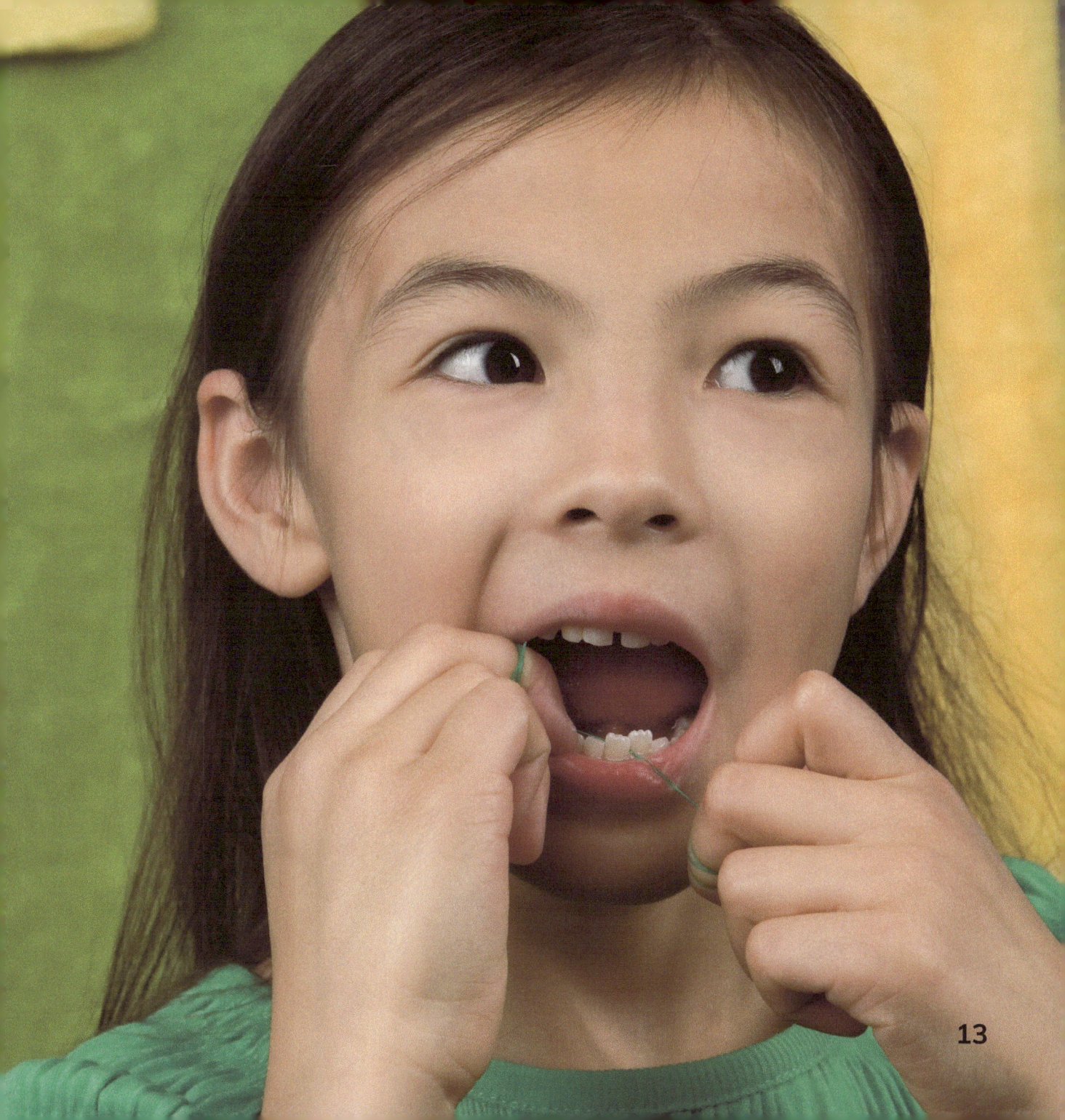

Going to the Dentist

It's important to go to the **dentist** two times a year. Why? A dental **hygienist** will clean and polish your teeth. They will floss your teeth too.

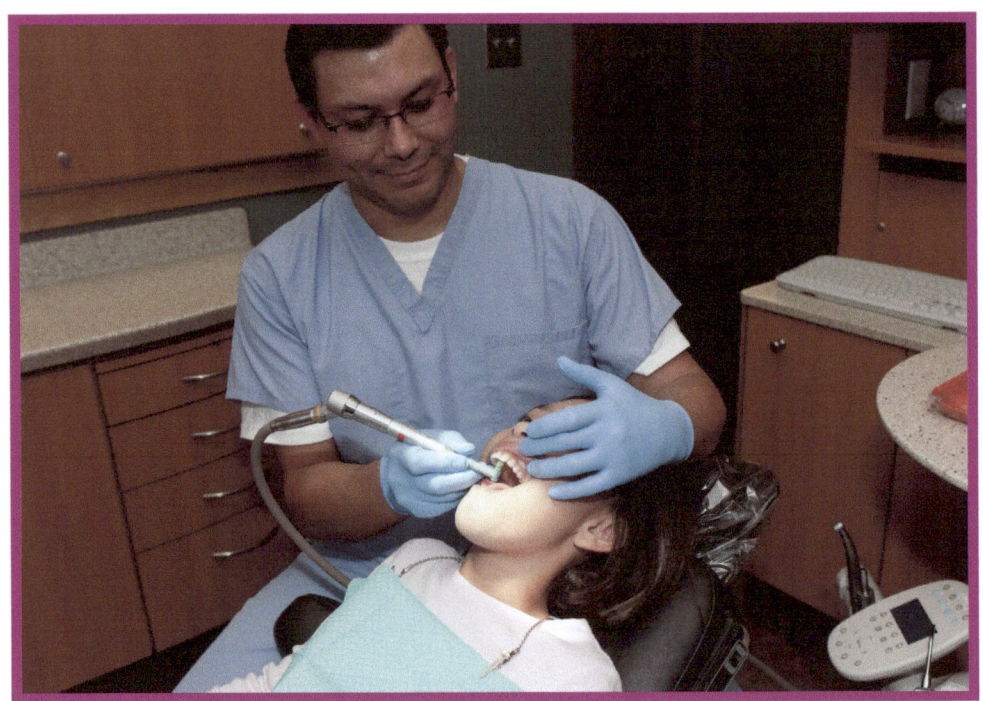

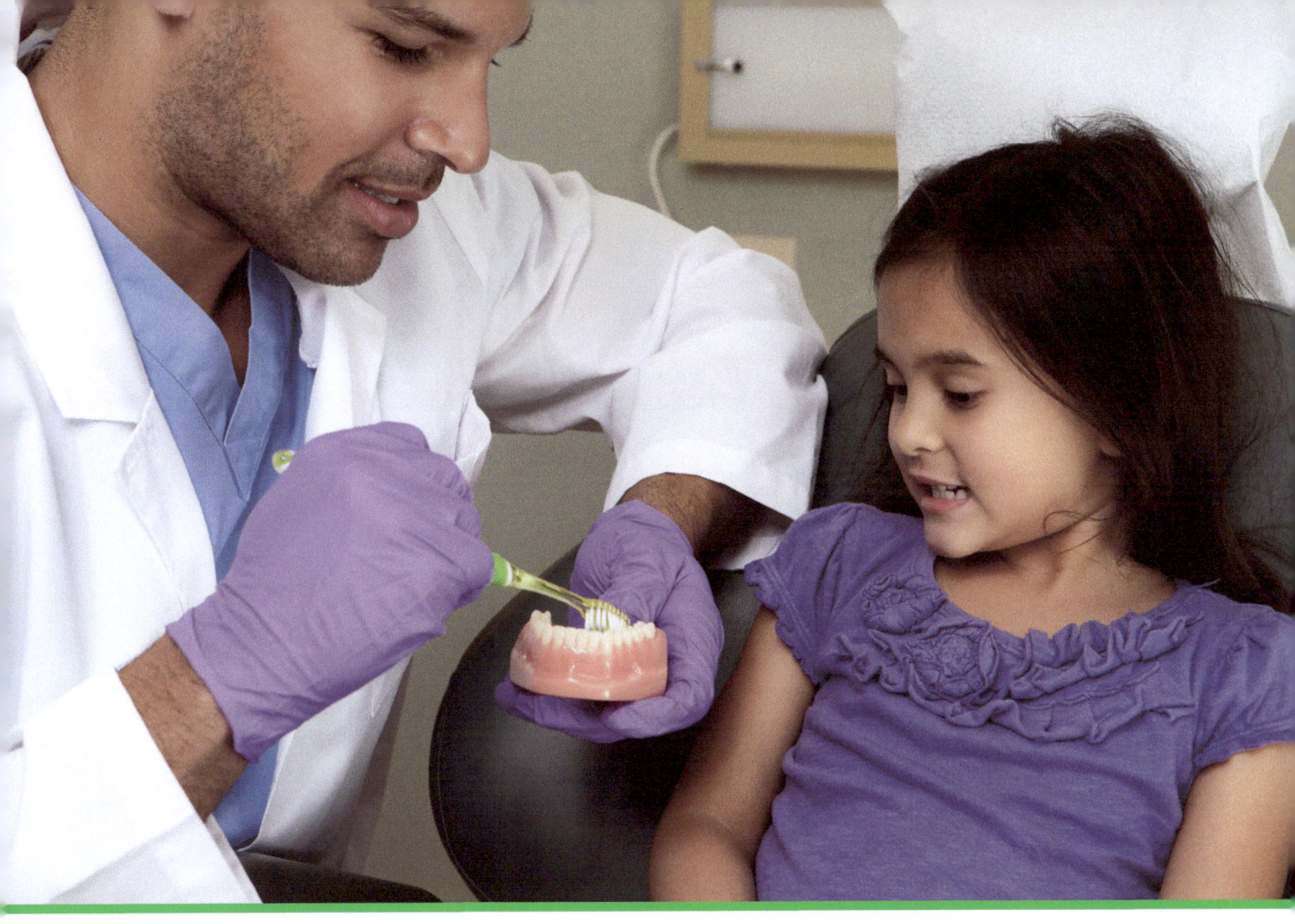

The dentist checks your teeth and gums. They look at **X-rays** of your teeth. They look for cavities or other problems. The dentist might show you the best way to brush.

Healthy Eating

Healthy foods build strong, healthy teeth. Be sure to eat fruits and vegetables each day. Eat cheese, yogurt, and nuts too. Drink water every day.

Sweets, juice, and soda have sugar. Too much sugar is bad. It can cause tooth decay and cavities. So enjoy sugary food and drinks once in a while. They can be a treat. Then rinse your mouth or brush your teeth.

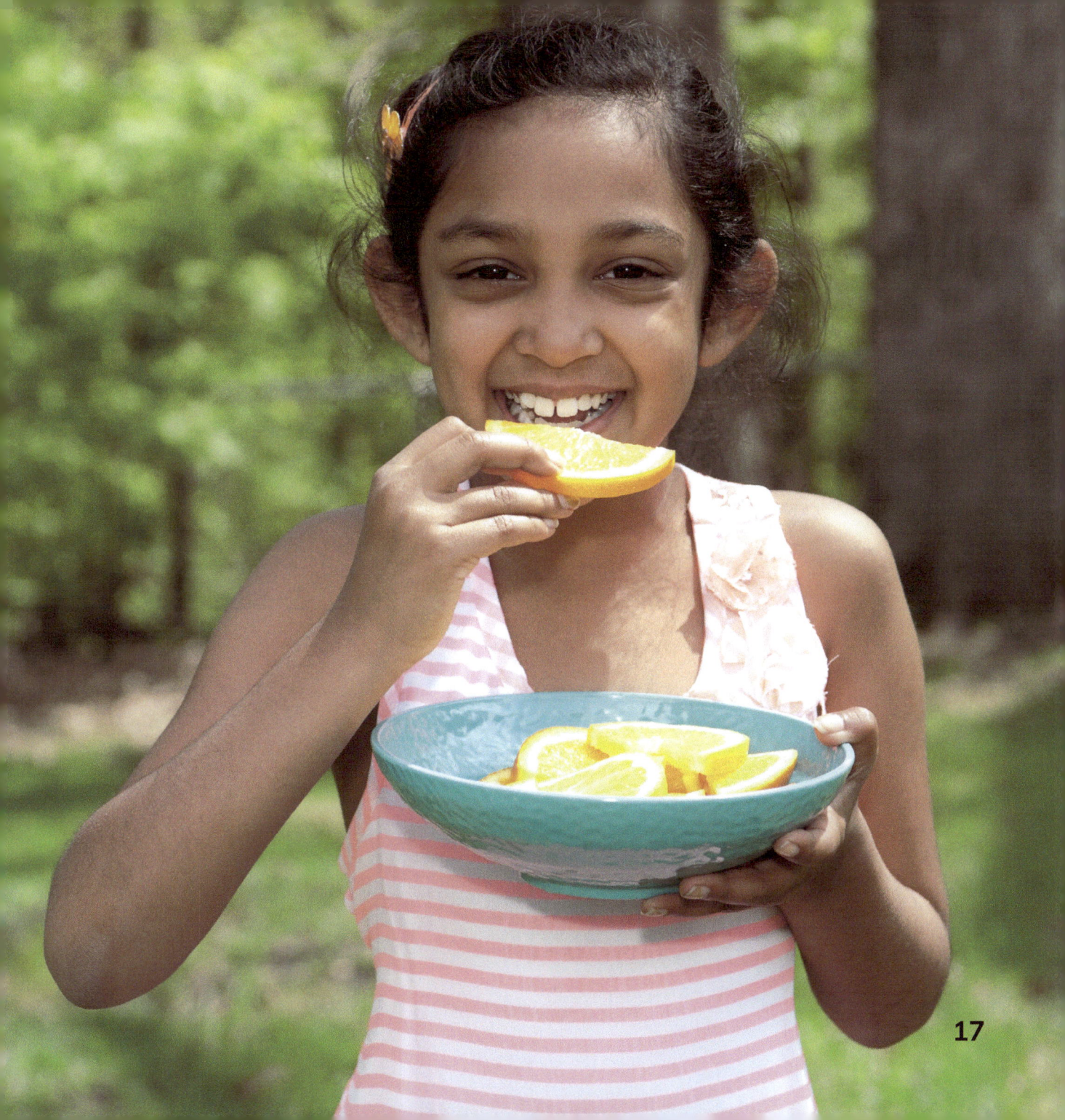

Make It a Habit

It's important to care for your teeth every day. Make it a **habit**! Take your time. Do not rush. Use a calendar to keep track of when you brush. Add a fun sticker each day.

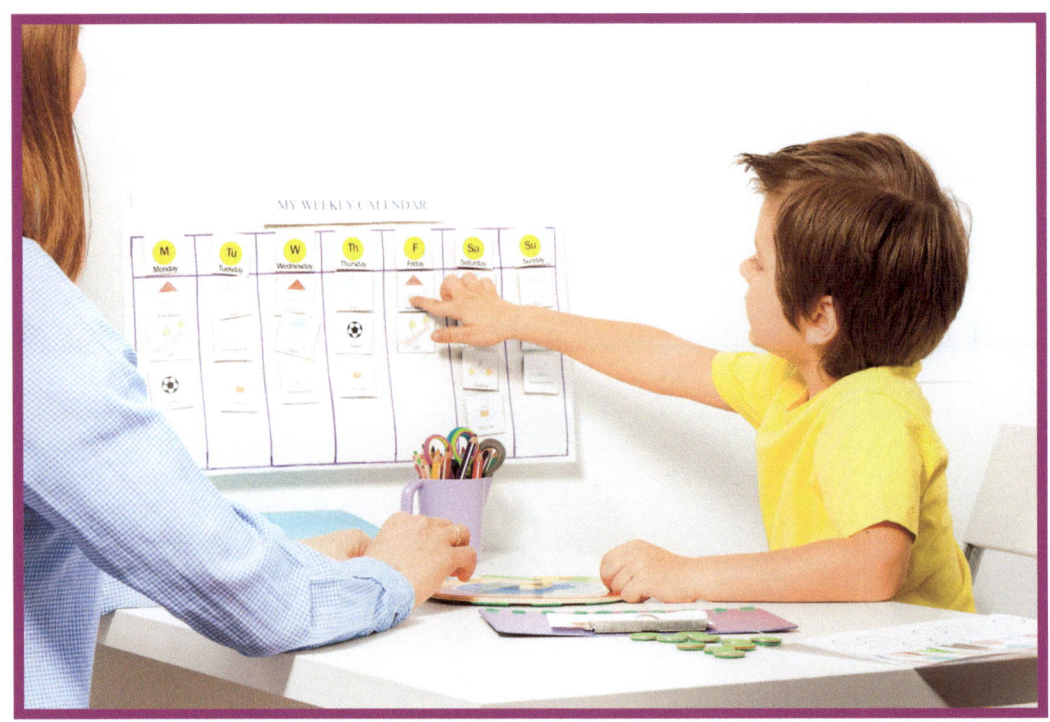

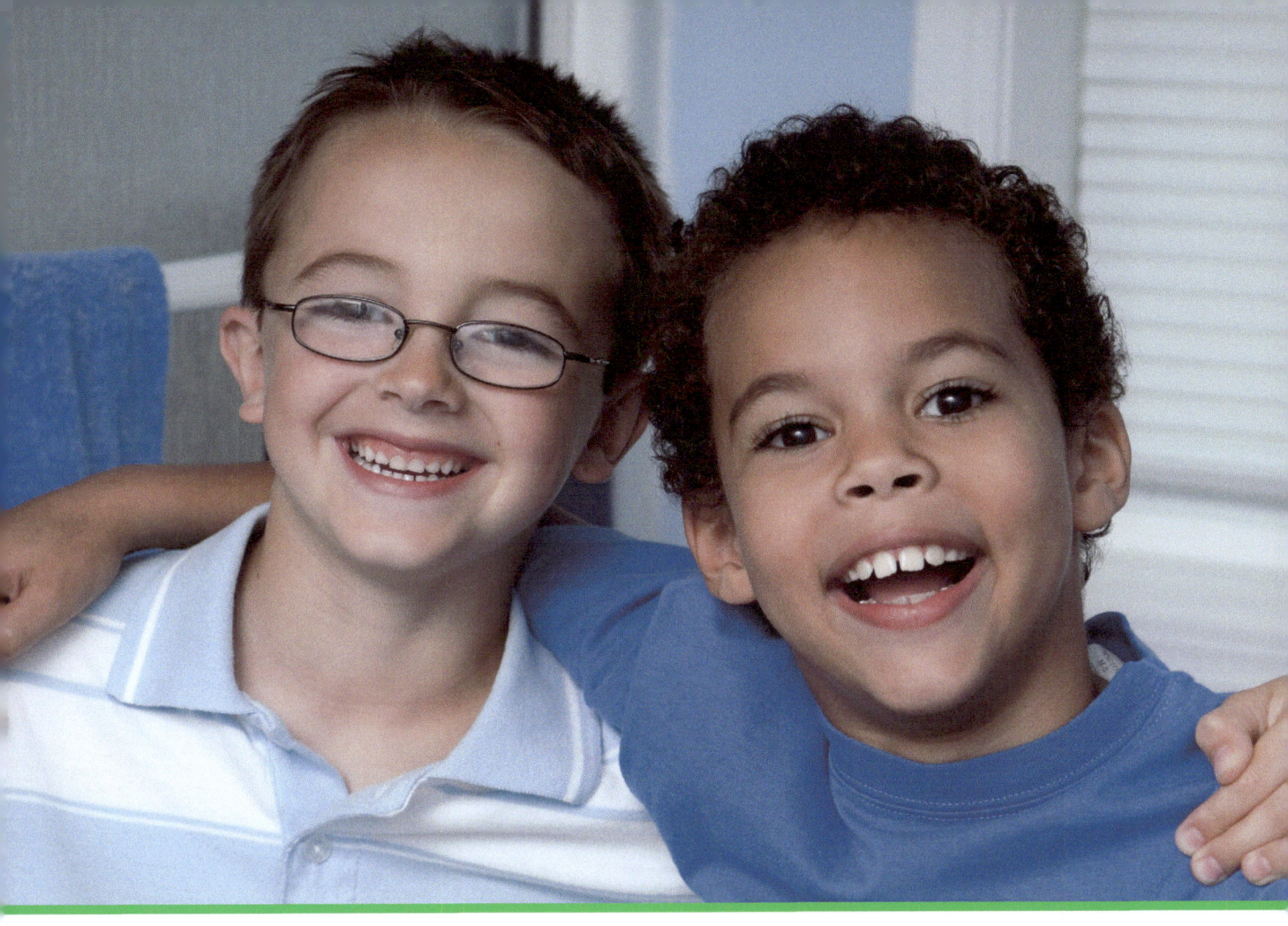

Set a **goal** to take good care of your teeth. Then you will have strong teeth. You will have a bright, healthy smile.

Egg in Soda

Sugar can harm your teeth. Try this activity to see why brushing your teeth is a healthy habit.

What You Need:

- 2 hard-boiled white eggs with the shells on
- 2 clear cups
- water
- dark soda, such as root beer or cola
- toothpaste
- toothbrush

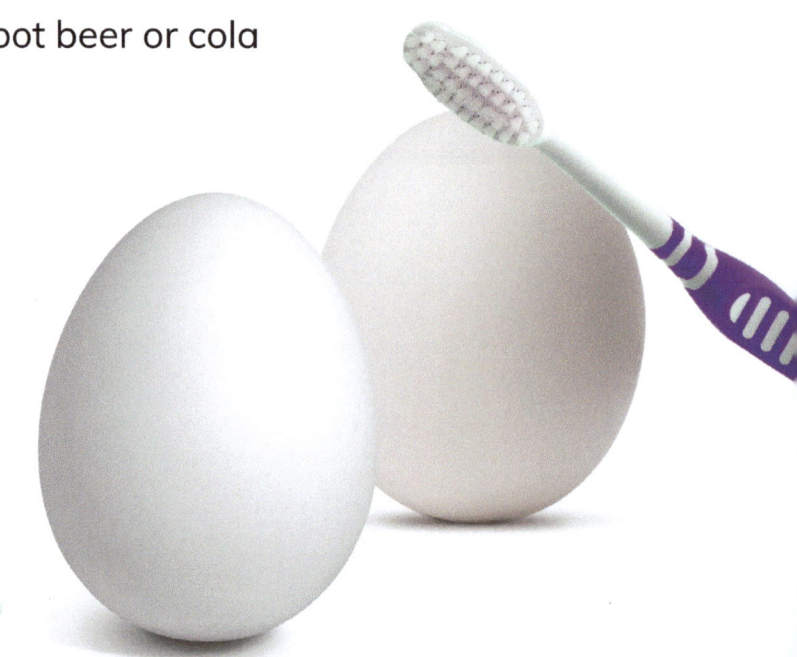

What You Do:

1. Put one egg into each cup.
2. Pour water into one cup. Pour soda into the other cup.
3. Keep the eggs in the cups overnight.
4. Look at the eggs the next day. Do they look the same? Or do they look different?
5. Use toothpaste and a toothbrush to clean the egg that was in the soda cup. How long does it take for the stain to come off?

The eggs are like our teeth. Our teeth can be harmed by sugar. Our teeth need to be carefully brushed to stay healthy and clean.

Glossary

cavity (KAH-vuh-tee)—a hole in a tooth caused by rotting

dentist (DEN-tist)—a person who is trained to check, clean, and fix teeth

floss (FLAWS)—a thin thread used to clean in between teeth

fluoride (FLOOR-yd)—a natural mineral that is applied to teeth to make them stronger and help prevent cavities

goal (GOHL)—something that you aim for or work toward

gum (GUHM)—the firm flesh around the base of a person's tooth

habit (HAB-it)—something that you do often

hygienist (hye-JEN-ist)—a person who is trained to help a dentist; hygienists clean teeth and take X-rays

plaque (PLAK)—the coating of food, saliva, and bacteria that forms on teeth and can cause tooth decay

X-ray (EKS-ray)—a picture taken of the inside of the body that can show if something is wrong

Read More

Jenkins, Pete. *Brush Your Teeth!* Vero Beach, FL: Rourke Educational Media, 2019.

MacReady, R.J. *Going to the Dentist.* New York: Cavendish Square Publishing, 2022.

Marsico, Katie. *Floss Your Teeth!* Ann Arbor, MI: Cherry Lake Publishing, 2019.

Internet Sites

American Dental Association: Oral Health Made Easy
mouthhealthy.org/en/resources/activity-sheets/oral-health

KidsHealth: What's a Cavity?
kidshealth.org/en/kids/cavity.html

Index

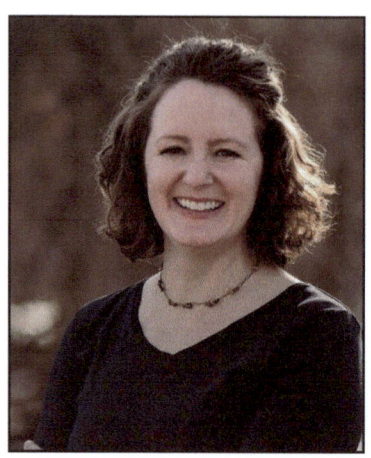

About the Author

Mari Schuh's love of reading began with cereal boxes at the kitchen table. Today, she is the author of hundreds of nonfiction books for beginning readers. Mari lives in the Midwest with her husband and their sassy house rabbit. Learn more about her at marischuh.com.